How to Manage Dementia at Home

Overcome caregiving challenges with this insightful guide

Jaylen Fleming

All right reserved. No part of this publication may be reproduced, stored in a retrieval system, or transmitted, in any form or by any means, electronic, mechanical, photocopying, recording or otherwise, without prior permission.

This book is sold subject to the condition that it shall not, by way of trade or otherwise, be lent, re-sold, hired out or otherwise circulated without the publisher's prior consent in any form of binding or cover other than that in which it is published and without a similar
condition including this condition being imposed on the subsequent purchaser.

Copyright©2024 by Jaylen Fleming

OTHER BOOKS BY SAME AUTHOR

- POST SEPSIS SYNDROME : Practical PSS Management Guide - Jaylen Fleming

- SEPSIS SYMPTOMS HANDBOOK : How to know if you have sepsis or not - Jaylen Fleming

- POST SEPSIS SYNDROME : Health after sepsis, healing after sepsis - Jaylen Fleming

- DEMENTIA FOR DUMMIES: A comprehensive self - aid guide with over 40 questions and answers - Jaylen Fleming
- ADHD and Women's Success - Jaylen Fleming

TABLE OF CONTENT

Introduction

Chapter 1
Understanding dementia

Chapter 2
Adapting the home environment to promote safety and independence
-Safety tips for around the home
-Implementing memory aids and reminders
-Establishing routines and consistency

CHAPTER 3
Tips for improving communication with individuals with dementia
-Ways to communicate with a person with dementia

Chapter 4
Practical tips for assisting with daily tasks
- Why daily activities and routines are important for people with dementia
- Activities for people with dementia at home
- Day-to-Day Routine Improvements

Chapter 5
Addressing nutrition and hydration needs for dementia patients
- Coping with changing eating habits
- Managing overeating

Chapter 6
Strategies for managing caregiver stress and burnout
- Tips to manage caregiver stress
- Get the appreciation you need

-Applaud your own effort

Conclusion

About the Author

Introduction

As a seasoned clinical professional specializing in dementia care, I've had the privilege of witnessing the complexities and nuances of this condition firsthand. Every day, I've encountered individuals and families grappling with the profound impact of dementia on their lives. From the initial diagnosis to the progression of symptoms, the journey is fraught with challenges, uncertainties, and moments of profound resilience.

Through years of experience, I've come to understand that while dementia may present formidable obstacles, it also offers opportunities for growth, compassion, and profound connection. It's within the context of these experiences that I've crafted this comprehensive guide on managing dementia at home.

Drawing upon both my professional expertise and personal insights, this book aims to provide practical strategies, empathetic support, and valuable resources for those navigating the complex terrain of dementia care within the familiar confines of home. Whether you're a caregiver seeking guidance, a family member seeking understanding, or an individual living with dementia seeking empowerment, this book is designed to be a beacon of knowledge, reassurance, and hope.

Join me as we embark on a journey of understanding, resilience, and compassionate care. Together, we can navigate the challenges of dementia with grace, dignity, and unwavering dedication.

Chapter 1

Understanding dementia

In a quaint little town nestled amidst rolling hills and winding rivers, lived my eccentric uncle Harry. With his bushy eyebrows, mischievous grin, and penchant for colorful

Hawaiian shirts, Uncle Harry was the life of every party and the source of endless laughter. Little did we know that beneath his jovial exterior, a silent storm was brewing.

It all began with the curious case of the missing keys. One sunny afternoon, Uncle Harry burst into the kitchen, his eyes wide with panic.

"Has anyone seen my keys? I swear I left them right here on the counter!" he exclaimed, frantically rummaging through drawers and pockets.

My aunt, ever the voice of reason, calmly reassured him that his keys were probably just hiding in plain sight. But as the days went by and the keys remained elusive, we began to suspect that something more than absent-mindedness was at play.

As weeks turned into months, Uncle Harry's forgetfulness became more pronounced. He would forget where he put his glasses, his wallet, even his own name on occasion (though he always laughed it off as a senior moment). But it was his obsession with the refrigerator that truly raised eyebrows.

"Have you seen my sandwich? I could have sworn I left it in the fridge," he'd declare, only to discover it in his hand or halfway eaten on the sofa. The fridge became a symbol of both mystery and comedy in our household, as Uncle Harry waged a daily battle against its perplexing contents.

One fateful morning, as Uncle Harry stumbled bleary-eyed into the kitchen, he was greeted by an unexpected sight: his toaster was talking to him.

"Good morning, Harry! How about some toast to start your day?" the toaster chirped cheerfully.

Uncle Harry blinked in disbelief, then burst into laughter. "Well, I'll be darned! Who knew toasters could talk?"

From that day on, the talking toaster became Uncle Harry's loyal companion, dispensing words of wisdom (and the occasional burnt slice of toast) with unwavering enthusiasm.
As Uncle Harry's dementia progressed, his grasp on reality began to loosen. He would regale us with tales of his daring exploits as

a young man – sailing the seven seas, taming wild beasts, even journeying to distant planets.

"Did I ever tell you about the time I rode a unicorn through the streets of Paris?" he'd declare, his eyes sparkling with mischief.
We'd exchange knowing glances and play along with his fantastical stories, knowing that in Uncle Harry's world, anything was possible.

Despite the challenges of dementia, Uncle Harry never lost his sense of humor. He greeted each day with a smile, finding joy in the simple pleasures of life – a warm cup of tea, a friendly game of cards, the company of loved ones.

And so, as we navigated the twists and turns of Uncle Harry's grand adventure, we discovered that laughter truly is the best medicine. In the face of adversity, humor became our greatest ally, shining a light in the darkest corners of dementia and reminding us that even in the midst of chaos, there is always room for laughter and love.Though Uncle Harry's journey with dementia was filled with ups and downs, it was also a testament to the power of laughter, resilience, and the indomitable human spirit. And though he may have forgotten many things along the way, he never forgot the joy of a good joke or the warmth of a loving embrace. As we bid farewell to Uncle Harry and his unforgettable antics, we carry with us the laughter, the love, and the enduring legacy of a life lived with humor and grace.

- Asking the same question over and over again or forgetting recent events

are signs of dementia. For example, even though they were told about a family member's visit just moments earlier, they can still inquire about it.
- Even easy things like making a grocery list or following a recipe might become difficult. They could have trouble keeping track of the steps or become disoriented in the middle.
- People could forget the passing of time, the seasons, or the dates. Even in familiar circumstances such as their own house, people may experience disorientation and forget where they are.
- Dementia can lead to agitation and mood swings, which are frequently brought on by bewilderment or frustration. For instance, losing track of a familiar object or having their

routine interrupted can make someone agitated.
- Some individuals with dementia may wander aimlessly, driven by a sense of restlessness or disorientation. They may leave the house without warning, putting themselves at risk of getting lost or injured.
- Sundowning is the term used to describe the increased disorientation, agitation, or anxiety that some persons with dementia experience as nighttime draws near. For caregivers, this might cause sleep habits to be disturbed and make evenings especially difficult.
- Basic activities like bathing, dressing, and grooming may become difficult to manage independently. A person with dementia may forget how to perform these tasks or resist help from

caregivers due to feelings of embarrassment or frustration.
- Dementia is characterized by communication problems that impact both spoken and nonspoken interactions. I had worked with a woman whose dementia progressed to the point that she had trouble understanding other people's words and expressing herself coherently. The patient struggled to communicate their needs and feelings to caregivers and loved ones, which resulted in frustration and isolation.

Dementia affects individuals of all genders, yet there are notable differences in how the condition manifests and progresses between men and women. Understanding these nuances is crucial for providing tailored care and support. Here's a glimpse into the uniqueness of dementia in different genders:

- Compared to men, women are more prone to get dementia. According to certain research, women may have a higher incidence because they often live longer lives. Cognitive performance and the risk of dementia may be impacted by menopause and hormonal changes in women. It has been suggested that estrogen protects the brain, which may postpone the onset of dementia symptoms in women.

- Compared to men, women with dementia may present with distinct symptom patterns. Although memory loss is a typical early symptom for both sexes, women may be more severely affected by verbal memory impairment and linguistic challenges. Women with dementia may experience behavioral and psychological symptoms such social disengagement, anxiety, and depression more frequently.Men who have dementia may behave impulsively, aggressively, and agitatedly more frequently.

1. Research suggests that the underlying pathology of dementia may differ between men and women. For example, Alzheimer's disease, the most common form of dementia, may progress differently in men and women, with women potentially experiencing more rapid cognitive decline.Vascular risk factors such as

hypertension, diabetes, and cardiovascular disease may have a stronger association with dementia in memen.

2. Women are more likely than males to become a person with dementia's primary caregiver, frequently juggling caregiving duties with other responsibilities to their families and their jobs. Increased stress, burnout, and caregiver load may result from this. Men may be less likely than women to seek help or support when dealing with dementia-related issues, which could delay diagnosis and prevent them from receiving the right treatment and resources.

3. It's critical to provide therapies and support services that are specifically

designed to meet the requirements and preferences of both men and women with dementia. Gender-specific support groups, caregiver education initiatives, and culturally competent care methodologies are a few examples of this. Men and women have received the same pharmacological treatments for dementia, such as memantine and cholinesterase inhibitors, yet there may be disparities in the side effect profiles and treatment response between the sexes.

CHAPTER 2

Adapting the home environment to promote safety and independence

A dementia patient's ideal living situation is one that promotes their maximum level of independence and happiness. It's crucial to be familiar with the surroundings because changes could make people more confused and disoriented. Your house should be a place that helps you figure out who you are and where you want to go.

Safety tips for around the home

Electrical
- Make sure the lighting is optimal by drawing the curtains and blinds, using high-wattage lightbulbs, and using sensor lighting to sense when a person enters the space.
- To help with nighttime navigation to the restroom, install nightlights in the restroom and halls. Remove electric blankets and hot water bottles as they may pose a safety risk.
- Automatic cut off for hot water jugs and other appliances are recommended

- Replace more dangerous forms of heating, such as bar radiators, with safer heating options like column heaters
- Check appliances, such as heaters and toasters, to make sure they do not present any safety hazards
- Replace long electrical cords on appliances with coiled or retractable cords.

Bathroom and other rooms

- Hand held shower hoses allowing to direct the flow of water as desired
- A shower or bath seat so you can be seated while bathing and eliminates the need to lower yourself into the bath
- Install hand rails at the bath, shower and toilet

- Arrange furniture simply and consistently and keep the environment uncluttered
- Remove loose rugs and seal carpet edges that may be safety hazards
- Make sure mats are secure that patterns in flooring are minimal
- Dispose of (or safely store) all medications
- Smoke detectors are important for everyone. A person with dementia may need someone to check the battery and make sure the alarm is loud enough
- If you live alone, consider a device or system that will alert someone if you are unwell or have left the home
- Consider security cameras inside and outside the home that are connected to an app that track movement

- Set up an engaging environment with magazines and jigsaws
- Ensure items to complete activities are in easy sight i.e. teabags, coffee and sugar or tea towels for drying dishes.

In the garden

- Keep paths well swept and clear of overhanging branches
- Check catches on gates and consider padlocking gates with word and number combinations
- Remove poisonous plants and dispose of hazardous substances from sheds and garages such as kerosene.

In the Kitchen

- The kitchen can be a hazardous place for people with dementia, but there are ways to make it safer and easier to navigate.

- Keep cups, teabags and other frequently used items on the kitchen counter
- Replace solid cupboard doors with clear doors so the person can see what's inside, or stick lists or photographs of the contents to the doors
- If possible, install taps that are clearly marked 'hot' and 'cold' or if this isn't possible, write the words on labels beside the taps
- Check use-by dates regularly and discard anything that is out of date

- Consider buying independent living aids such as adaptive chopping boards, can/jar openers, graters, etc
- Keep toxic cleaning products in a locked cupboard
- Speak to the gas supplier about installing a gas valve limiter – these are usually free, and prevent gas hobs being turned on accidentally or left on
- Use a flood and scald protection plug in the sink – these change colour if the water is too hot, and automatically drain the water once it gets to a certain depth if the tap is left running. They are available from shops selling.

In the Living Room

- Living rooms should be relaxing and cosy, so ensure chairs and sofas are comfortable and offer good support. Assistive furniture, which helps people stand up and sit down more easily, can be very useful – although sometimes expensive.

- The living room is one of the most common places where falls happen, but you can take steps here and throughout the home to reduce the risk.

- Remove rugs, or make sure the edges are stuck down
- Keep the floor clear of clutter, especially trailing wires
- Check that the person's slippers and shoes fit properly
- Keep essential objects like glasses and remote controls in a set place, within easy reach

- Take away electric fires or heaters that could be accidentally left on or tripped over
- Remove furniture with thin legs that could be tripped over
- A personal alarm that the person can press if they fall may offer reassurance – these are usually worn on a lanyard
- Although many people enjoy having the TV or radio on, try to avoid leaving them on if the person is no longer watching or listening. Background noise or sudden loud noises can cause confusion and distress, which could lead to accidents. You can buy simple remote controls with large, clearly labelled buttons that work with any television.

In the Bathroom

Many people with dementia have problems with vision and how they perceive objects, colours and patterns, which can cause confusion in the bathroom.

It may help to:

- stick a written sign or a picture of a toilet to the door to help the person locate the bathroom
- fit a coloured toilet seat that is a different colour from the toilet itself, so it's easy to see
- use coloured toilet paper on a freestanding holder
- choose brightly coloured towels so they stand out on the towel rail

Other steps to make the bathroom safer include:

- keeping the toilet lid up
- leaving the light on at night
- removing toilet and bathmats, so that the person doesn't slip on them
- installing grab rails at useful points around the bathroom
- using flood and scald prevention plugs

Implementing memory aids and reminders

- Labels and signs can be quite helpful if the person with dementia has trouble remembering where things are kept or how their home is laid out.

- Avoid introducing too many signs at once to avoid overloading the person. Start with the ones that would be most beneficial. For example, you might label the refrigerator with images of milk and cheese or place a picture of a toilet on the door of the bathroom.

- Signs ought to be readable, clear, and at eye level. You can purchase signs from assistive living stores or download and print graphics from the internet.

- If the person with dementia has memory problems, you could try:

- hanging a whiteboard somewhere conspicuous to write reminders of appointments, events, visitors etc

- displaying a large 'dementia clock' which shows not just the time, but also the day, date and time of day (ie morning, afternoon, evening, night)
- setting audible reminders on the person's phone or smart speaker, but only if you are sure they will not be distressed or confused by them.

Establishing routines and consistency

People who have dementia may experience confusion and chaos every day. With all of their additional duties to assist their loved ones, caregivers frequently feel overburdened.

In the absence of proper planning, concern, medication, and baths consume the days. You can, however, regain some degree of control. By incorporating routines, you can help reduce their anxiety and restore a semblance of regularity to both of your lives.

Why Do Routines Help in Dementia Care?

People living with Alzheimer's disease and other forms of dementia lose short-term memory first, making it more difficult to accomplish daily tasks and keep track of where and when they are.

Long-term memory persists far into the middle and late stages of the illness, despite the short-term memory decline. This is something that both of you and they can profit from.

When routines are followed consistently, they become automatic and are stored in long-term memory. Your loved one will become more independent and you will be relieved of some of their burdens if you establish routines and habits together.

Reasons to Create a Routine

You'll find no downside to establishing routines as part of your dementia care plan. Incorporating them as soon after the diagnosis as possible will be the most beneficial for both of you.

(1) Maintain Skills

If someone doesn't use a talent, they can lose almost any ability, especially if they have dementia. If the patients with the illness don't routinely use their abilities, they quickly forget them.

Establishing a regimen in which they take showers, brush their teeth, put on clothes, and perform other necessary tasks at least somewhat autonomously aids in the maintenance of those abilities. If not, you will have to take over basic tasks as their caregiver when they become unable of performing them themselves.

(2)   Reduce Caregiver Load

The majority of caretakers struggle to prioritize their own needs and frequently put the needs of their loved ones before their own. But you have to look after yourself. When you're angry and exhausted, you won't be a nice person for them. Establishing a schedule where kids finish specific duties on their own will allow you to take a few minutes to unwind.

While they brush their teeth or while they take a bath, you may read a chapter of a book or watch their favorite TV show on your phone. While it makes sense to remain alert and close by, you'll have a little more breathing room if you're not as physically involved.

(3) Keep Them More Independent

For those with dementia, especially those who are accustomed to being active or living alone, losing their freedom can be quite difficult. Your loved one might even act out and resent your assistance in the early and middle phases of the illness. They will feel independent once more if you assist them in creating a routine and involve them in it. They will have a little more autonomy and be able to do more things on their own.

(4) Lessen Patient Anxiety

For those who require additional structure in their lives, routines and habits are crucial. Being more present and reducing anxiety are achieved by having a daily routine.

Dementia patients experience the same thing. They have trouble remembering who is next to them, where they are, and what day it is. Extreme dread and anxiety are the result of all these problems together, yet a routine is comfortable and can help reduce worry.

What Does a Dementia Care Routine Look Like?

The regimen for dementia care need to resemble your loved one's existence before dementia as much as feasible. If they already followed a morning or evening routine, starting now will increase the likelihood that they will continue it as the illness worsens.

You might organize your day around important daily chores, morning and nighttime activities, or the entire day. Making a daily routine will act as a reminder to change things up and offer chances for relaxation, exercise, and stimulation. All those necessary elements should be included in a well-rounded strategy.

8 Tips for Creating a Routine for Dementia Patients

How do you create a routine for your loved one with dementia? What do you need to know to set up an effective schedule? Let these tips help you establish the ideal plan.

(1) Give Them a Say

It's best to start soon after their diagnosis or on a lucid day. This way, your loved one can help you create a schedule that fits their interests and desires. It will also give them a sense of control when everything else seems chaotic and unfamiliar.

(2) Watch Their Patterns
If their condition is advanced to the point where they can't help you create a routine, try to remember any they may have had before their diagnosis:

Can you recall any portions of their morning or evening regimens?
When you started taking care of your loved ones, did they have preferences for doing certain tasks and specific times of the day?
Any commonalities you can keep will encourage them to adhere to the schedule and bring a sense of calming familiarity.

(3) Include Exercise

Exercise is a critical component of any dementia patient care plan. It's a mood booster and stress reducer that can improve brain function, decreasing the rate of memory loss.

Physical activity increases the number of dendrites in each neuron. The dendrites connect to other neurons in the brain, and more connections mean improved recall, problem-solving and decision-making.

(4) Focus on Repetition

Completing the same tasks in order every day can give patients with dementia a sense of control. They know what will happen, so they have something to look forward to and expect. Even when everything else feels out of control, they have a tried-and-true routine to ground them.

(5) Incorporate Fun Activities
Repetitive routines are important, but you should occasionally change up your loved one's activities, offering new and fun alternatives to keep their mind and body active. One could be Memory Joggers to challenge and strengthen recall.

If you plan the whole day, set aside a few different time slots to rotate through their favorite pastimes, like taking a walk, chatting with friends, gardening or reading.

(6) Remember Rest
Patients with advancing dementia may get tired more quickly than they used to. Plan rest breaks after any strenuous or exciting activities so they can recuperate. Otherwise, they'll grow overtired and get irritable and difficult to manage.

You could also get a much-needed break while they relax or sleep.

(7) Remain Flexible

Your loved one's needs and abilities will change day to day. It's important to keep the regimens as consistent as possible, but sometimes you must be willing to make changes.

They may require more rest one day or have a lucid moment and want to take advantage. Go easy on yourself and them by allowing some wiggle room within the routine.

(8) Add Essential Tasks

At the bare minimum, you'll want to create a schedule addressing all the essential daily tasks like brushing teeth, bathing, combing hair, getting dressed and so on. Processes like these can become automatic if repeated often enough.

Keep Them Home Longer With Routines
In the late stages of the disease, most people with dementia decline to the point where their caregivers can't take care of them independently. You'll need to hire a nurse to help or move them into a residential care facility.

However, if you integrate routines early on in their condition, the habit will keep them independent enough and prolong their time at home.

CHAPTER 3

Tips for improving communication with individuals with dementia

Dementia affects everyone differently so it's important to communicate in a way that is right for the person. Listen carefully and think about what you're going to say and how you'll say it. You can also communicate meaningfully without using spoken words.

Before you communicate:
- Make sure the person is comfortable

Make sure you're in a good place to communicate. Ideally it will be quiet and calm, with good lighting. Busy environments can make it especially difficult for a person with dementia to concentrate on the conversation, so turn off distractions such as the radio or TV.

If there is a time of day where the person is able to communicate more clearly, try to use this time to ask any questions or talk about anything you need to.

Make the most of 'good' days and find ways to adapt on more difficult ones.

Make sure any of the person's other needs are met before you start – for example, ensuring they are not in pain or hungry.

Preparing to communicate with a person with dementia

Think about how you might feel if you struggled to communicate, and what would help.

Plan enough time to spend with the person. If you feel rushed or stressed, take some time to become calmer beforehand.

Think about previous conversations you have had with the person and what helped you to communicate well then.

If the person has begun to communicate using the first language they learned, and you do not speak it, consider arranging for family members or friends who also speak the language to be there with you. If the person prefers reading, try using translated written materials. A translation or interpretation app on a smart phone or tablet can translate between you if you don't speak the same language. If you need an interpreter, speak to your local authority, the person's care home, or an organisation such as the Institute of Translation and Interpreting.

- Get the person's full attention before you start.

Things to consider about conversation topics

Think about what you are going to talk about. It may be useful to have an idea for a particular topic ready.
If you are not sure what to talk about, you can use the person's environment to help – anything that they can see, hear or touch might be of interest.
Listening

Tips for listening to a person with dementia
- Listen carefully to what the person is saying. Offer encouragement both verbally and non-verbally, for example by making eye contact and nodding.

This 'active listening' can help improve communication.

The person's body language can show a lot about their emotions. The expression on their face and the way they hold themselves can give you clear signals about how they are feeling when they communicate.

If you haven't fully understood what the person has said, ask them to repeat it. If you are still unclear, rephrase their answer to check your understanding of what they meant.

If the person with dementia has difficulty finding the right word or finishing a sentence, ask them to explain it in a different way. Listen and look out for clues. If they cannot find the word for a particular object, ask them to describe it instead.

- Supporting the person to express themselves

Allow the person plenty of time to respond – it may take them longer to process the information and work out their response.

Try not to interrupt the person – even to help them find a word – as it can break the pattern of communication.

If the person is upset, let them express their feelings. Allow them the time that they need, and try not to dismiss their worries – sometimes the best thing to do is just listen, and show that you are there.

Ways to communicate with a person with dementia

- Use short, simple sentences.

Don't talk to the person as you would to a child – be patient and have respect for them.

Try to communicate with the person in a conversational way, rather than asking question after question which may feel quite tiring or intimidating.

Include the person in conversations with others. It is important not to speak as though they are not there. Being included can help them to keep their sense of identity and know they are valued. It can also help them to feel less excluded or isolated.

If the person becomes tired easily, then short, regular conversations may be better.

- Avoid speaking sharply or raising your voice.

How to pace conversations

Go at a slightly slower pace than usual if the person is struggling to follow you.

Allow time between sentences for the person to process the information and respond. These pauses might feel uncomfortable if they become quite long, but it is important to give the person time to respond.

Try to let the person complete their own sentences, and try not to be too quick to assume you know what they are trying to say.

- Things to consider about body language

Stand or sit where the person can see and hear you as clearly as possible – usually this will be in front of them, and with your face well-lit. Try to be at eye-level with them, rather than standing over them.

Be as close to the person as is comfortable for you both, so that you can clearly hear each other, and make eye contact as you would with anyone.

Prompts can help, for instance pointing at a photo of someone or encouraging the person to hold and interact with an object you are talking about.

Try to make sure your body language is open and relaxed.

What to communicate
- Tips for asking questions

Try to avoid asking too many questions, or asking complicated questions. The person may become frustrated or withdrawn if they can't find the answer.

Try to stick to one idea at a time. Giving someone a choice is important, but too many options can be confusing and frustrating.

- Phrase questions in a way that allows for a simple answer. For example, rather than asking someone what they would like to drink, ask if they would like tea or coffee. Questions with a 'yes' or 'no' answer are easier to answer.

What to do if the person has difficulty understanding
Try explaining what you're saying in a slightly different way if, despite your repeated attempts, the other person still doesn't comprehend. If the recipient is having trouble understanding, you might want to explore dividing your message into more manageable bits.

- Try to laugh together about misunderstandings and mistakes. Humour can help to relieve tension and bring you closer together. Make sure the person doesn't feel you are laughing at them.

Chapter 4

Practical tips for assisting with daily tasks

"All too often, we as caregivers struggle to manage the emotional and behavioral toll dementia can take on the person for whom we care. People with dementia often struggle with depression, isolation, lethargy, and loneliness. This can lead to challenging behaviors like wandering, withdrawal, and agitation," says Saran Craig, Senior Clinical Implementation Specialist at Careforth.

"In my 10 years working with people with dementia, I have found that engaging in simple activities with the person with dementia is one of the best therapies and one of the greatest tools for dementia caregivers!"

Everyone enjoys different activities, so it's vital to locate the ones that best fit the personality and lifestyle of the person getting care. This will help you choose which activities to include in your caregiving routine. It's crucial to comprehend the effects that involvement and activity can have on a dementia patient's quality of life and general wellbeing.

Why Daily Activities and Routines are Important for People with Dementia

All older persons should follow a daily schedule that includes healthy activities, but those who have dementia or other cognitive impairments should prioritize it even more. As dementia worsens, the individual will become increasingly disoriented and have trouble picking up new skills.

For individuals who are still in the early stages of the disease, routine gives them a sense of control over their day and surroundings. Many of these activities are frequently the only means by which people with end-stage dementia can continue interact with their memories and communicate.

Additional benefits of incorporating engaging activities in one's daily routine include:

- Stimulating Cognitive Function: Staying active helps keep the mind engaged and ready for new experiences and can be used to maintain social bonds which can aid in memory recall and improve wellbeing.
- Providing a Source of Focus: By organizing events and getting together frequently, friends and family can offer structure. Adding consistency to a person's daily routine might help

lower stress levels and provide a focal point for a person suffering from dementia.
- Building a Feeling of Productivity: Many people who suffer from dementia believe that they are a burden to their loved ones. Small or large, daily tasks can give one a sense of success and productivity.
- Advice from Careforth Care Team: Make sure not to engage in any activities that could cause your loved one too much stress or challenge. Establishing a good atmosphere is crucial before adding new activities to a person's daily schedule.

Activities for People with Dementia at Home

By keeping them engaged in meaningful activities and active, a few recommendations from Careforth's trained care teams can help improve the quality of life for both the dementia patient and the caregiver. Throughout all stages of dementia, there are many methods to make positive changes in one's life. These include rearranging one's daily routine, engaging in creative pursuits like music and art, playing cognitive games, exercising, and going outside. Consider taking these steps to begin your journey toward improved health and wellness.

Day-to-Day Routine Improvements

Adding additional duties and activities to your daily routine is one of the simplest ways to increase activity to your life. Take into consideration these ten possibilities for activity to get you started on the right path of improving your daily routine:

- Visit somewhere familiar and pleasant.
- Create daily activities to mimic their former work life.
- Eat and sleep at the same times each day.
- Don't be afraid to talk about the past. Consider this: Reminiscing can reduce symptoms of depression, improve communication, boost self-esteem,

and reconnect someone with their family history and memories.
- Spend time sorting and organizing.
- Get a fish tank or aquarium. Consider this: Introducing a large fish tank in a person's dining area can increase appetite and weight gain in residents with dementia.
- Try pet therapy or adopt a furry friend.
- Cook or bake together.
- Indulge in aromatherapy.
- Use community resources.
- Music and Art Projects
- Arts and crafts, as well as music, can be incredibly powerful for those with cognitive disabilities and can be an excellent way to connect. Consider these 10 expert tips:

- Listen to music together, and don't be afraid to sing along. Consider this: Music has been shown to help people with dementia feel calmer, improve their mood, create social connections, and slow the decline of cognitive function.
- Keep a journal tracking daily activities and exercising memory recall.
- Create a box filled with photos and memory-filled objects.
- Take dance breaks.
- Try knitting or crochet.
- Get crafty or pick up a paintbrush. Consider this: Using art as a form of therapy can reduce stress, anxiety, and depression, and can play a critical role in facilitating engagement and social connections for those with dementia and other cognitive illnesses.
- Take a stroll around a museum.

- Play with modeling clay to help with dexterity.
- Make your own musical instruments.
- Read a book together. Consider this: According to a 14-year study, reading activity can prevent long-term decline in cognitive function in seniors.
- Brain Games for Dementia

As dementia progresses, many cognitive skills – like arithmetic, counting, memory recall, etc. – become difficult and distressing. Games and apps focused on strengthening and exercising these cognitive skills can be a great source of mental activity for someone with dementia. Examples of brain games and activities include:

- Play cards and board games.
- Solve daily crosswords and jigsaw puzzles.

- Use comedy and improvisation to bring laughter to your day and live in the moment. Consider this: According to Mayo Clinic, laughter can reduce stress, improve your immune system, relieve pain, and improve your mood and outlook.
- Play brain-training or word game apps.
- Play with dolls or toys.
- Get Active and Exercise

For people with dementia, staying active and getting outside are vital to keeping a person engaged in everyday life. To accomplish this, try integrating daily or weekly activities outdoors, at local community centers, or in your own neighborhood. For inspiration, consider the following activities:

- Dig in the garden.
- Take a dip in the local pool.
- Go for a walk through the neighborhood.
- Try chair exercises fit for seniors with varying physical abilities.
- Unlock the power of mindfulness through yoga and massage therapy. Consider this: Physical touch – such as hand or foot massages – has been shown calm agitated behaviors, reduce stress, and ease physical discomfort.
- Taking Action to Improve Your Loved One's Wellbeing – A Closing Invitation

"Often the old activities that brought the person we care for meaning, purpose and joy are not possible. A common cause of depression, withdrawal, or challenging behaviors in someone with dementia is lack of activity and purpose. To put it in the simplest terms – they're bored!" says Craig. "If you're experiencing emotional or behavioral challenges with the person you care for, you might find introducing activity is your solution! Introducing new, simple activities to a person with dementia will not only brings them joy and meaning, but it will also give you a simple tool to connect, improve quality of life, and enhance relationships."

When it comes to providing care for someone with a chronic illness or disease, you don't have a do it alone.

Chapter 5

Addressing nutrition and hydration needs for dementia patients

The primary cause of people's inadequate nutrition and hydration is their problems with swallowing, eating, and drinking. Eating and drinking can be more challenging for individuals with dementia due to memory loss and physical challenges, even though maintaining a good, balanced diet is crucial. The following are some problems that may arise as a result of confusion and dementia:

- Forgetting about their eating routine, leading to potential overeating.
- Missing meals.
- Eating the same food daily.
- Experiencing difficulties in preparing food or drink.

The primary cause of people's inadequate nutrition and hydration is their problems with swallowing, eating, and drinking. Eating and drinking can be more challenging for individuals with dementia due to memory loss and physical challenges, even though maintaining a good, balanced diet is crucial. The following are some problems that may arise as a result of confusion and dementia:

(1) Helping people with Dementia to drink

The relationship between dementia sufferers & drinking is their inability to recognise when they are thirsty or knowing how to communicate their thirst. Here are some tips below on how to encourage those to increase their fluid intake .

Always having a drink next to the person, put it where they can see it clearly.
In case they dislike water, provide them with hot or cold beverages or add some flavor. If they have trouble holding the glasses, assist them in drinking. Urge the person to consume foods like gravy, yoghurt, and ice lollies that are high in liquid. assisting the elderly in eating Encouraging those with dementia to eat mostly involves ensuring their comfort. Being flexible with mealtimes is one of the best things you can do to help someone eat more leisurely. The setting of where they are

dining can also be beneficial. You can make sure the space is well-lit and turn off any loud distractions, such the radio or TV. Additional suggestions consist of:

(2) Be led by the person with dementia on where they would like to sit and eat. Ensure that they are comfortable.

Serve meals in moderation; avoid piling too much food on the platter. To prevent hot food from getting cold and losing its charm, think about serving half quantities. Get them involved in preparing dinner. It might encourage them to eat if you and the others are eating at the same time. If they have trouble swallowing, consult your doctor. Dementia-related weight gain or decrease Dementia-related eating and drinking disorders might put patients at risk for malnourishment and weight loss. They might also have weakness and fatigue.

(3) Make food look and smell appealing. Use different tastes, colours and smells to stimulate their appetite.

Give the person gentle reminders to eat, and remind them what the food is.

If they don't want to eat a main meal at set times, try preparing finger food to snack on instead

Overeating is a massive risk with sufferers being drawn to sweet or starchy foods and forgetting that they have recently eaten. Whilst making sure they do not gain an unhealthy amount of weight you should look to replace the sweet/starchy food with healthier alternatives, for example fruit or low-calorie jelly. Other solutions towards overcoming weight gain can include:

(4) Serving food in smaller portions.

Ensure that the person has something to do, so that they don't feel bored or lonely.

Make sure the person is well hydrated as they may be mistaking thirst for hunger.

Consider not having certain foods in the house, or substituting them with low-fat or low-calorie versions.

Changes in eating habits and food preferences

Sometimes people with dementia make food choices that don't match their usual beliefs or preferences. For example, a person who has been a lifelong vegetarian may want to eat meat for reasons including:

- their preference has changed

- they remember that they used to eat meat (before they became vegetarian)
- they have forgotten they don't eat meat
- they see you or someone else eating meat and want the same, without knowing what it is.

For similar reasons, people who have other beliefs may start to want something different that they previously wouldn't have eaten. For example, a person who does not eat pork for religious reasons may start to want pork. It can be difficult to know what to do in these situations.

Read Lucy's experience of eating and drinking

Lucy's mum, Rosemary, is living with Alzheimer's disease. Here, Lucy shares the challenges they had with eating and trying to keep her mum safe in her own home for as long as possible.

Coping with changing eating habits

If a person has a preference for sweet foods, fruit or naturally sweet vegetables may be a healthier option if the person isn't losing weight. Adding small amounts of honey or sugar to savoury food can also help.
- Use herbs and spices, sauces and chutneys to enhance flavours.
- Add small amounts of syrup, jam or honey to puddings to increase sweetness.

- Be led by the person on what they'd like to eat, even if the food combinations seem unusual.
- Be led by the person on when they prefer to eat. Some people like a light lunch and larger evening meal and others prefer a main meal in the middle of the day. This may be different to when they've previously wanted to eat.
- Try food the person has never eaten before but remember the person's personal preferences and practices. Their beliefs should be respected despite changes in eating habits.
- Try to use what you know about the person and, if they're showing a different preference, consider what might be the reason for this.

Also be aware of any impact on the person's digestion. For example, if the person has always been vegetarian but asks for meat, offer meat substitutes instead. These may be easier for them to digest.

Always try to do what's in the person's best interests, even if this is different to the best interests of those around them.

Managing overeating

Some individuals suffering from dementia could not remember when they last had food or worry about when they will next be fed. A person who is overindulging may also consume inappropriate foods. They may be inquiring or looking for meals on a regular basis. Both them and the others around them may find this to be a stressful scenario.

Individuals suffering from specific forms of dementia, such frontotemporal dementia, might be more prone to binge eating and other alterations in their eating habits. Changes in dietary preferences and food obsessions are two examples of these. Excessive alcohol consumption is another risk factor for dementia.

Ways to help manage overeating
- Ensure that the person has something to do, so that they don't feel bored or lonely.
- Divide the original portion into two and offer the second one if the person asks for more.
- Fill most of the plate with salad or vegetables.
- Make sure the person is well hydrated as they may be mistaking thirst for

hunger. Ensure they have a drink with their meal if possible.
- Leave bite-sized fruit or healthy snacks, such as chopped bananas, orange segments or grapes, within reach for the person to snack on when they want to.
- Offer the person a low-calorie drink instead of more food.
- Consider not having certain foods in the house, or substituting them with low-fat or low-calorie versions.

If the person has developed a strong preference for particular foods, and is not eating enough of other foods, or if they are struggling with excess weight gain, ask the GP for referral to a dietitian.

Meal preparation

People with dementia who live alone may struggle to prepare meals, or may forget about food, which then goes off. This can have a bigger impact on their wellbeing if there's no other support in place to help them with these issues. If the person is struggling with eating and drinking, it may be a sign they need more support.

Supporting someone who is living alone

Urge the person to eat meals that are ready at room temperature, chilled, or frozen. They may make cooking easier for the person and frequently require minimal preparation. There are meals that are designed to be nutritionally balanced. Ready-prepared or frozen veggies can be a quick and simple approach to support someone who struggles to chop or peel vegetables to consume a balanced diet. Think about ordering takeout. In certain localities, there is a "meals on wheels" service. The individual might also be able to order premade meals for a week to be delivered. To find out what is available in your region, get in touch with your local council.

Organise online shopping if the person struggles with going to the shops. It can be a good way to make sure there is fresh food in the house. The person can order what they want and have it delivered – usually on the date and at the time of day that they choose. Others (such as friends or family members) could help the person with this, but it's important to make sure the food ordered is what the person would want.

Leave simple notes or pictures to show the person where food is – for example a picture of a sandwich on the fridge.

Chapter 6

Strategies for managing caregiver stress and burnout

Anyone who assists someone in need is considered a caretaker. An elderly friend or relative, a disabled child, or an ailing spouse or partner can all be considered those in need. While rewarding, providing care may be stressful. Providing care can be quite rewarding. It feels nice for most caregivers to take care of a loved one. It can also strengthen your relationship. However, the responsibilities of providing care often lead to physical and mental strain. Feelings like rage, frustration, exhaustion, or sadness are prevalent. It's also normal to feel isolated. Stress among caregivers can increase their chance of experiencing changes in their own health. Among the things that can make caregiver stress worse are:

- Caring for a spouse.
- Living with the person who needs care.
- Caring for someone who needs constant care.
- Feeling alone.
- Feeling helpless or depressed.
- Having money problems.
- Spending many hours caregiving.
- Having too little guidance from health care professionals.
- Having no choice about being a caregiver.
- Not having good coping or problem-solving skills.

- Feeling the need to give care at all times.

Signs of caregiver stress

As a caregiver, you may be so focused on your loved one that you don't see how caregiving affects your own health and well-being. The signs of caregiver stress include:

- Feeling burdened or worrying all the time.
- Feeling tired often.
- Sleeping too much or not enough.
- Gaining or losing weight.
- Becoming easily irked or angry.
- Losing interest in activities you used to enjoy.
- Feeling sad.

- Having frequent headaches or other pains or health problems.
- Misusing alcohol or drugs, including prescription medicines.
- Missing your own medical appointments.
- Too much stress over time can harm your health. As a caregiver, you might feel depressed or anxious. You might not get enough sleep or physical activity. Or you might not eat a balanced diet. All of these increase your risk of health conditions, such as heart disease and diabetes.

Tips to manage caregiver stress

Even the most resilient individual can become exhausted from the mental and physical strain of providing care. You can look after yourself and your loved one with the aid of a lot of tools and resources. Utilize them. You cannot care for anyone else if you do not take care of yourself.

To help manage caregiver stress:

- Ask for and accept help. Make a list of ways in which others can help you. Then let them choose how to help. Ideas include taking regular walks with the person you care for, cooking a meal for you and helping with medical appointments.

- Focus on what you can do. At times, you might feel like you're not doing enough. But no one is a perfect caregiver. Believe that you're doing the best you can.
- Set goals you can reach. Break large tasks into smaller steps that you can do one at a time. Make lists of what's most important. Follow a daily routine. Say no to requests that are draining, such as hosting meals for holidays or other occasions.
- Get connected. Learn about caregiving resources in your area. There might be classes you can take. You might find caregiving services such as rides, meal delivery or house cleaning.
- Join a support group. People in support groups know what you're dealing with. They can cheer you on and help you solve problems. A

support group also can be a place to make new friends.
- Seek social support. Stay connected to family and friends who support you. Make time each week to visit with someone, even if it's just a walk or a quick cup of coffee.
- Take care of your health. Find ways to sleep better. Move more on most days. Eat a healthy diet. Drink plenty of water.

Many caregivers have trouble sleeping. Good sleep is important for health. If you have trouble getting a good night's sleep, talk to your health care professional.

See your health care professional. Get the vaccines you need and regular health screenings. Tell your health care professional that you're a caregiver. Talk about worries or symptoms you have.

Respite care

It may be hard to leave your loved one in someone else's care. But taking a break can be one of the best things you do for yourself and the person you're caring for. Types of respite care include:

- In-home respite. Health care aides come to your home to spend time with your loved one or give nursing services or both.
- Adult care centers and programs. There are centers that give day care for older adults. Some also care for young children. The two groups might spend time together.

- Short-term nursing homes. Some assisted living homes, memory care homes and nursing homes accept people who need care for short stays while caregivers are away.

Working outside the home

Caregivers who work outside the home can feel burdened. If this describes you, think about taking a leave from your job for a time if you can afford to do so.

Get the appreciation you need

Giving care can have daunting and draining duties. However, there are actions you can take to reduce stress and restore equilibrium, happiness, and hope in your life. Although taking care of a loved one can be immensely fulfilling, there are a lot of stressors involved. Furthermore, because providing care is sometimes a lifelong endeavor, the emotional toll can mount up over time. You could have to provide care for others for years or even decades. It can be especially depressing if you think you're overextending yourself, if there's little chance your loved one will recover, or if, in spite of your best efforts, their condition is steadily getting worse.

Unmanaged caregiver stress can have a negative impact on your relationships, health, and mental state. Ultimately, it can cause burnout, which is characterized by emotional, mental, and physical tiredness. And when that happens, it hurts you and the person you're taking care of as well. Because of this, looking after yourself is essential rather than optional. Ensuring your loved one arrives at their doctor's appointment or takes their prescription on time is not as vital as taking care of your own physical and mental health. Stress can generally feel overpowering, but burnout is more akin to long-term tiredness. You may go from saying things like "I have too much on my plate" to "I'm done" if you've reached burnout.

Avoid caregiver burnout by feeling empowered.
Feeling powerless is the number one contributor to burnout and depression. And it's an easy trap to fall into as a caregiver, especially if you feel stuck in a role you didn't expect or helpless to change things for the better. But no matter the situation, you aren't powerless. This is especially true when it comes to your state of mind. You can't always get the extra time, money, or

physical assistance you'd like, but you can always get more happiness and hope.

- Practice acceptance: Making sense of the circumstance and asking "Why?" is frequently necessary while dealing with the injustice of a loved one's illness or the responsibility of providing care. However, you can expend a lot of energy worrying about things that you cannot alter and for which there are no satisfactory solutions. You won't feel any better at the end of the day either. Aim to stay away from the emotional pitfall of looking for someone to blame or feeling sorry for yourself.

- Embrace your caregiving choice: Recognize that you have chosen to give care consciously, despite any grudges or responsibilities you may have. Consider the advantages of such decision. Maybe you give care to make up for the nurturing you received from your parents when you were a child. Or perhaps it has to do with your morals or the example you wish to provide for your kids. These profound, significant drives can support you throughout trying times.

- Take an organized approach: As a caregiver, you might be responsible for keeping track of important medical and legal papers, medications, and appointment dates. When items get lost or dates get mixed up, feelings of powerlessness can quickly creep in. Use binders to organize paper documents and folders on your computer to maintain digital information. A calendar or planner can help you remember when it's time for doctor visits and prescription refills

- Look for the silver lining: Think about the ways caregiving has made you stronger or how it's brought you closer to the person you're taking care of or to other family members.

- Don't let caregiving take over your life: Since it's easier to accept a difficult situation when there are other areas of your life that are rewarding, it's important not to let caregiving take over your whole existence. Invest in things that give you meaning and purpose whether it's your family, church, a favorite hobby, or your career.

- Focus on the things you can control: You can't wish for more hours in the day or force your brother to help out more. Rather than stressing out over things you can't control, focus on how you choose to react to problems.

- Break big tasks down into manageable chunks: Thinking about all the caregiving tasks you need to complete this week, for example, can make you feel overwhelmed or uncertain about where to start. Instead, make a to-do list for each day and begin to work through it one task at a time.

- Celebrate the small victories: If you start to feel discouraged, remind yourself that all your efforts matter. You don't have to cure your loved one's illness to make a difference. Don't underestimate the importance of making your loved one feel more safe, comfortable, and loved!

Applaud your own effort

Being acknowledged goes a long way toward increasing one's ability to enjoy life and to tolerate a difficult circumstance. Research indicates that caregivers who feel valued have better mental and physical health. Despite its demands, providing care really makes them happier and healthier. What would you do, though, if the person you are taking care of is unable to express or feel gratitude for your time and efforts?

If your loved one were well, picture their reaction. How would your loved one feel about the love and care you're providing if they weren't concerned with their health or suffering, or if dementia prevented them from functioning? Remember that if the other person could, they would convey their gratitude.

Praise your own initiatives. If you're not receiving approval from others, find methods to appreciate and treat yourself. Remind yourself of the extent of your assistance. Try compiling a list of all the ways your caregiving is improving things if you require something more tangible. Go back to it whenever you're feeling down. Speak with a friend or family member who is encouraging. It's not necessary for the person you're taking care of to provide positive encouragement. Seek support from friends and family who will listen to you and recognize your efforts if you feel undervalued.

Conclusion

Managing dementia at home is undoubtedly challenging, but with the right knowledge, support, and resources, it is possible to create a nurturing and fulfilling environment for both individuals with dementia and their caregivers. This book aims to empower you with the tools and strategies needed to navigate this journey with compassion, resilience, and hope.

About the Author

Hi, I am Dr. Jaylen Fleming. With over 10 years of clinical experience, I am a seasoned publisher dedicated to providing compassionate self-help resources on human health issues and diseases to patients and other health practitioners. Follow me for updates, and get my books to keep yourself enlightened and liberated.

Follow me on Amazon author central to get more of my books
https://www.amazon.com/author/drjaylen1